Family First
A Road Map to Private Elderly Health Care
Written by: Charlotte Mullaney

This workbook is intended to give those who are in the position of finding personal care for their ageing loved ones a complete "road map" in a simple, efficient and user-friendly format. This guide has been developed from my professional experience and research and is not intended to give you any legal or financial advice. It will guide you and help you create a thorough and effective "what you need to know" to coordinate care for your loved ones.

I managed a private home health care staffing agency. After leaving the agency I wondered why people go with an agency for private care. Agencies are the "middle men" and on average, they double the per-hour cost than a private aide would be compensated. Why don't people find their own private care? The reasons are usually quite simple, "you don't have resources, the need is urgent, you don't know where to start, what to consider, what to watch out for, how to coordinate the care provider and services". In short, the main reason is that it is too overwhelming on top of what you have in your own personal lives: kids, jobs, crucial commitments. I intend to show you that finding, coordinating and maintaining your own private care is possible by following these tips and insights.

Topics for Consideration:

1. Identifying active participants
    a. Care scheduler/manager
    b. Care receiver/patient
    c. Care provider/care giver
2. Responsibilities
    a. How, what, and to whom responsibilities should be allocated
3. How you find an aide and managing reasonable expectations
    a. How to find an elderly healthcare aide
    b. How to develop your schedule
    c. How to successfully introduce an aide and implement a schedule
    d. How many hours you need and how many aides you should consider hiring accordingly
    e. How to protect everyone if there is a difficult experience
    f. How to pay an employee
    g. Forms to consider and prioritize based on family requirements
    h. Handbook example

*Every other page is left blank for your NOTES. I urge you to do this as you read through, not after the fact. Your first "ah-ha" moment pertaining to your instincts regarding this topic is usually your best. It also helps when/if you are combining these notes with your siblings' notes. What has been common between all or most of you? This is something that needs consideration as you map out a plan for caring for an elderly loved one.

Notes:

A few statistics to consider while you read this:

Here is a reality check: MA agency's hourly rate ranges from $19.00 - $26.50 per hour. The national mean hourly rate for CAN (Certified Nurse's Aide)/HHA (Home Health Aide) in 2012 was $12.32 per hr, here's a quick hourly, to weekly to monthly breakdown of cost savings: private vs. public...

Between 2012 – 2022 the home health care industry is predicted to grow 48%

* *US Dept. of Labor: Bureau of Labor Statistics:*
http://www.bls.gov/oes/current/oes311014.htm#nat
www.bls.gov/ooh/health-aides.htm

Schedule	~ Example mean rate from independently surveyed MA agency's $19 - $26.50 per hr. Mean rate: $22.75 per hr.	~ National mean hourly rate in 2012 was : $12.32 per hr.	Savings *Not including fed/state tax deductions
1 hr.	$ 22.75	$ 12.32	$10.43
10 hrs.	$ 227.50	$ 123.20	$104.30
20 hrs.	$ 455.00	$ 246.40	$198.60
30 hrs.	$ 682.50	$ 369.60	$312.90
40 hrs.	$ 910.00	$ 492.80	$417.20
50 hrs.	$ 1,137.50	$ 616.00	$ 521.50
60 hrs.	$ 1,365.00	$ 739.20	$ 625.80
70 hrs.	$ 1,592.50	$ 862.40	$730.10
80 hrs.	$ 1,820.00	$ 985.60	$ 803.60
90 hrs.	$ 2,047.50	$ 1,108.80	$938.70
100 hrs.	$ 2,275.00	$ 1,323.00	$952.00
110 hrs.	$ 2,502.50	$ 1,355.20	$1,104.70
120 hrs.	$ 2,730.00	$ 1478.40	$1,251.60
130 hrs.	$ 2,957.50	$ 1,601.60	$1,355.90
140 hrs.	$ 3,185.00	$ 1,724.80	$1,460.20
150 hrs.	$ 3,412.50	$ 1,848.00	$1,533.50
160 hrs.	$ 3,640.00	$ 1,971.12	$1,668.88
168 hrs.	$ 3,822.00	$2,069.76	$3,822.00

Notes:

<u>**Keeping your sanity!**</u>

Step 1:
Organizing home health care can be a time consuming and overwhelming position. You not only have your own responsibilities, but you also need to create, execute and maintain care, and provide for an aging family member – unless you have a plan of action.
Execution of care is threefold: care receiver, caregiver and care scheduler.

A)   <u>Care receiver</u>: From my professional experience, I have found that most "cared for" say that the most difficult time in their life was when they had to rely on friends and family for simple requests. Most care recipients find it difficult when they are unable to continue with their day-to-day priorities or activities. People at the stage of needing a little or a lot of help are extremely vulnerable. I cannot stress enough how important it is for the family to understand the emotional tension associated with the removal of personal independence. Spending time with the care receiver and documenting the precise schedule and behaviors they have grown accustomed to (not what you feel their needs are and what the plan is) is vital in order to create a comprehensive Sunday – Sunday model for the care receiver in order for the plan to run as smoothly as possible.

- What are the habits? What are the emotional triggers? E.g.: some might like to be kept on a schedule, some might not like to be rushed to dinner, some might like to have a chit chat and some might rather the aide be seen but not heard, – all must be clearly defined in advance...smooth transition is what you're hoping for.
- It's also very important to keep the cared for in the know. The minute they think they are being 'duped' or left out of decisions an emotional wall goes up and it's even harder to introduce the possibility of care providers. If you force an aide on the care receiver, there is going to be a huge resistance, which ultimately will create obstacles, as you will have to put a lot more work into the acceptance and execution of care. Be upfront and respectful of the cared for's intelligence by incorporating them into all the decision-making. Be open to asking them what their priorities are as this will build their security and confidence and can only be of benefit.

B)   <u>Caregiver</u>: You want to make sure you staff to the best of your ability. You will staff wrong at some point...it's ok. Just like most people, some prospective employees might talk the talk but can then fail to walk the walk? Sometimes it's just not the right fit.
- Be thorough, don't rush an interview, and take note of language skills, of limiting schedules, transportation, past experiences and kindness. Most importantly, hire people that smile and have a positive disposition; a smile goes a long way. When you do find the aides you want and ones that the care receiver is comfortable with, make the environment as welcoming and commutative as possible.

C) <u>Care Scheduler</u>: assuming that you are taking the reins, initiate a family meeting immediately to discuss primary objectives for care.
- Have a clear definition of the pros and cons of personally scheduling care instead of going through an agency (time vs. money). Important considerations are keeping your loved ones in their home, saving money for the unknown, management of care providers, control of the care, keeping informed.
- Keep in mind that everyone MUST buy-in and take on a responsibility(s) in the coordination of care. If two of the three offspring are doing all the work, there will be animosity or resentment. Also keep in mind the greater good and that is your loved one.
- Really talk about what your personal schedule permits are and who can handle what load of care. Once the family agreement is structured, you should have a monthly family meeting to discuss what's going on, what needs to be reconsidered, which aide is a Family First aide and which aide might need to be replaced etc. E.g.: the family member responsible for reading the aide journal on a monthly basis might find it evident that one of the aides is not abiding by the care plan. All aides should respect the next person coming on duty and do their utmost to provide a consistent environment they would like to come into.

Notes:

Responsibilities:

Step 2:
Family/friends will have to step up to bat. If you want to be totally hands off finding and sustaining your loved one's personal care and doing this all yourself instead of going with an agency, this is not the route for you. As with anything, the beginning is the hard part, but if put together properly your 'care plan' will run smoothly; however, you will need to manage it like a small business. In fact, when a family or friend decides to find their own personal care, they should know that it will take consistent maintenance, re-evaluation and time. If you have a larger family and it's not just you coordinating this care, then you should have a 'family meeting' and <u>divvy up the responsibilities</u> to balance the responsibilities and agree on a point person to coordinate the members and track progress.

Who finds the aide/s (startup responsibility)?
Who manages the schedule, aides and payroll (weekly responsibility)?
Who manages the bills: groceries, petty cash etc. (weekly responsibility)?
-         Keep a weekly log for groceries, an envelope for bills that need to be picked up and paid, etc.
-         Keep a log of petty cash, what it was spent on, and the recipes should be initialed by the aide.
Who reads the journal and makes adjustments to the next month's calendar (doctor's appointments, church meetings etc.) and checks in to make sure things are rolling as they should?
Who coordinates all of the above to make sure it is being done, points persons for aides outside of the above perimeters and communicates between all of the responsibility holders?

What does your cared for need and want and who is responsible?

What is it?	Need / Want (yes / no)	What days	Who's responsible	Notes/tips
Home-delivered meals				Maybe you qualify for free or reduced cost delivery (meals on wheels). * A great option if there are dietary restrictions (low salt, liquid diets for swallow issues etc.). It takes the liability out of an aide or the cared for person preparing meals incorrectly or cooking at all.
Shopping assistance / Grocery list preparation				See if you know anyone who already has someone do their shopping and add onto it (saves you the trip and any confusion in the store). Or look into grocery stores that deliver, such as Stop and Shop's PeaPod service

Bathing				
Dressing				
Toileting				
Continence				Have adult pull ups available just in case of an emergency
Eating				
Transferring				One aide should never be responsible for the total weight of one person. If this is the case you need to look into mobile assistance (wheelchair to toilet sliders, handrail grips etc.)
Homemaker services				With some aides you may be able to add 'light housekeeping' to their job duties. However, be aware that in doing this you are taking the watchful eye off your loved one. In this case, if there is a fall etc. (especially if the cared for is on 24hr's) then it is not the aide's fault.
Laundry				
Cooking				
Home repairs				
Caregiver issues				
Help with medications				Medications are tricky. They have to be sorted by a nurse or family member into daily (AM/PM) dispensers that are clearly labeled. If the cared for refuses their medication they cannot be forced or tricked into taking it. Medication can be placed into the hand of the cared for or crushed for example in applesauce but the cared for has to be told they are receiving their medication. All medication should be documented in the notebook. If it is refused, the aide should inform the care-coordinator a.s.a.p.
Nursing services				A visiting nurse (VN) should be someone you have already identified in your area for questions and home visits when necessary.
Wound care				Can be administered by a CNA not a HHA without a release of liability signed. Wound care is very important as the elderly do not typically heal fast and skin is frequently very thin and prone to breaks. When starting wound care, all aides should be shown how to do this not just told.
Tube feeding				Tube feeding can be administered by an aide; however, changing of the tubes and cleaning are best administered by a nurse.
Catheter changing				Visiting nurse (to avoid infection)
Injections				Visiting nurse
Financial Management / Tax help				Have a CPA or accountant to work out the budgets.

Banking				You can have all checks (Social Security etc.) sent to the accountant and also have the accountant put money in a separate account that the person in charge of withdrawals (for petty cash etc.) has access to. This account should be online for everyone to see to avoid issues.
Bill paying				If you can pay bills online and give everyone access to viewing the bill payments it will alleviate a lot of headaches.
Insurance policy management/counseling				
Post office chores				
Legal help				Have a health care proxy set up.
Social Needs				Organizing visitors, social outings (church, bingo, bridge games etc.)
Telephone reassurance				
Postal alert program				
Escort/transport to doctor appointments				
Physical Activities				Massage, walking, light exercise etc.
Physical Therapy				
Medical alert system				
Mind activities				Cards, board games, puzzles, reading, movies
Movies				

This is a good jumping off point for your job description also.

Notes:

How do I find an aide, and then what do I need to do!?!

Step 3:
How do you find an aide?

Here is the bad news: my advice is NOT to get an aide from an agency for the 'time being' if possible. A connection will be made and then what are you going to say/do? If you have no option, what you want to ask for (believe it or not) is a different aide as much as possible, so that a connection cannot be made while you are finding full-time care and consistency of care. I know this sounds awful, and I would say family and friends should step in if possible to avoid this but if that is not an option (if there is bathing/personal care needs that are not appropriate or uncomfortable for family to perform), have a lot of different aides so the cared for cannot get attached and when you do find an aide to head the ship they will be well received and appreciated. A short-term solution is also elderly daycare while you are in the process of finding an aide/s. This 'in-between time is also a great opportunity to start putting together the care plan model.

Home health care and certified nurse's aides (CNA) training programs are a HUGE industry. Go online; look into aide training programs in your area (in your area is key because the aides in training most likely live close by, therefore, they will be more apt to jump in if someone calls out or if you need shorter hours). You call the local Red Cross number they will also have a list of programs in your area. When you find a few training/certification programs talk to the program administrators about their 'graduation' dates. Most training agencies will have a small ceremony that they are happy to have prospective employees attend. You can talk to the aides and see if anyone fits your model. You should also talk to the administrators about their credit classes (in the state of MA, aides need 12 hours of training annually to keep up their certifications). This way you will be able to 'poach' an aide who is seasoned. You could offer the training company a stipend/donation for their help – believe me it will be well worth it if you find an aide who is confident, trained and knows what to do, in opposition to finding one who is just starting out. Maybe put an advertisement in your local church's newsletter/bulletin board. Or simply go to websites such as www.care.com to look at who is looking for work in your area. Alternatively, do you know a neighbor or friend in the area who has an aide for their aging loved ones? Talk to them about inquiring with their aide if they know of anyone else who would be interested, or go to your local aging community center; they usually will have referrals or a bulletin board with aides' information. Do the footwork; collect as many names as possible.

Getting your schedule together:
Before you start posting for your aide or the interview process, you need to create your model.

Create a short bio/job profile of the most important traits (both professionally and personality wise) you need in an aide and for an aide to perform, as the first point of discussion to briefly outline your expectations and the work environment.

Think about the personality type of whom you need help for. Are they quiet? Are they particular? Do they love to be read to? Make sure you can understand the aide properly.

It's very important when dealing with the elderly the aide needs to be able to speak clearly to avoid frustration and miscommunication when given or taking direction. Do you

need your aide to cook meals? Do you need an aide who loves animals (in many cases there is a dog or cat that is the apple of the cared for eye – many people do not like animals (for some Haitian and African cultural there is a differential). Make sure you know that the care shown for the animal is satisfactory. Would it be wonderful if they had an interest in gardening or playing the piano? Define what makes up your loved one and the aide presented to them will be much better received than just someone who can do the job. In addition, the most
important thing to look for is an aide who smiles and is patient.

Beware of aides with tight schedules, children they need to pick up, drop off to school, no car, therefore reliant on someone else to transport them…there will be a day when you get a call that the aide has an emergency and has to leave or cannot come in, it will happen. When you are talking to your prospective aide, ask a lot of questions about their limitations. Start with a phone interview, then an interview in person, and then thirdly allow the aide to meet the client.

Notes:

How to successfully introduce an aide and implement a schedule:

  Introducing an aide is the most delicate situation. In the majority of cases, the cared for does not think they need it or want it. It is very important to spend time with the aide to show them exactly how things should be done. When I say exactly I mean it, I've had aides fired by clients because they don't brush their hair right, iron their clothes right, butter their toast to the edges, make their bed right, buy the wrong kind of milk etc.. In the beginning, any reason is a good one and the anxiety of the cared for person is at a peak because they are essentially giving up their independence, and a stranger is in their home – and no one wants that. If you put time in training and setting up very detailed guidelines, you have a much better chance of a solid working introduction and not having to repeat the process. You will also have someone who can train another person down the road. I have noted some lists that can be adapted to your situation but you should take what you need from these lists and make a checklist for the aide to follow. Routine is key. Consistency is key. Schedule is key. Checking in with both the aide and the cared for is key. The aide might tell you about forgetfulness or a symptom that you did not know about. The cared for in turn might tell you that the aide is talking on her phone or she was asleep during the night when called. What is working, what is not working? What needs to be changed and addressed. In the very beginning, getting this model down is detrimental. When setting up the chore schedule, be sure to do laundry the day you're cared for does laundry, empty the dishwasher when they do...make it like everything is the same. Always have the aide keep a detailed journal. Have the aide note exactly what was done on her shift on an hourly basis (not at the end of a shift). This is essential on many levels.

Most likely in the beginning you will need 2-3 hours in the morning (showering, dressing, breakfast, getting the paper, putting the laundry in, making a lunch putting it in the fridge etc.) and 2-3 hours in the evening (putting the laundry in the dryer, making dinner, undressing, going to bed etc.). Here is the trick: for fewer hours you will pay more, for more hours you will pay less. What will you pay? Depending on your location it can be anywhere from $8 an hour - $17 an hour, check your state income charts for more information on what home health care workers are making. If you are flexible, maybe you will get an aide who is looking for work after an overnight shift somewhere else or before a shift somewhere else. In general, an aide looking for full time work is looking for 12 – 24 hour shifts. If you need long hours, you are golden. All aides will want to work with you; you can even pay a salary rate (especially overnight if sleeping is allowed) rather than an hourly rate. You may even find an aide who will work 24 hours and that will be great for consistency but make sure the duties, especially if you need them awake during the night, are being done. Does your cared for refuse to call out in the night for help? Get an aide for the night shifts...avoid a fall at all costs. I know it sounds awful but a bell is usually a welcome tool for overnight shifts. There are of course devices like an alert mat – this is a mat put beside the bed so that when the cared for exits the bed it alerts the aide. Many people will think of bed rails, I have to say I disagree. It is a constraint and in case of an emergency it could be devastating.

Shift	# Of aides	Why
Mornings or Evenings	2	Alternate weekend mornings and offer coverage if someone needs a day off etc.
Both mornings and evenings (usually 2-3 hours each)	2-3: try to have the same aide do both shifts on alternative days	Because then all aides know both morning and evening routines.
Day shift (8-12 hours)	3-4	Longer day shifts are more likely to be harder to cover in a pinch. You want to have three aides in constant rotation and one as a backup for emergencies.
Night shift (8 – 12 hours)	2-3	Night shifts are in high demand and you will most likely have an easier time covering the shift. You also don't want too many shift changes as your aides want these shifts and will be happy to have a decent amount.
24 hrs.	5-6	Depending on your scheduling (independent contractor or salaried employee) you will want to divide up the hour so you do not run into overtime issues. You want to keep it a job rate. You can do 48-hour shifts once per week, therefore keeping the aide number down to 4 but be mindful that a 48-hour shift will be very difficult to cover in a pinch. However, the consistency of having the same person there and 'sleeping rates' can sometimes offset this if you have reliable aides.

Notes:

How do I protect everyone if something bad happens?

Step 4:

Protect yourself and your family from liability:

Unfortunately, there are some bad eggs out there and accidents happen. An aide may come in and slip and fall then sue you. Get umbrella liability insurance including workman's compensation. Get an inventory of assets and if possible keep a combination safe. Do your background checks and by this I do not mean call references, although of course you should do this also. I mean get a background CORI check on the aide (you can get the paperwork at your local police station and run an independent CORI check). The most common case of abuse is elderly abuse; cover your bases. If the aide is an independent contractor, make sure they really are (see the 20 questions that all ICs must adhere to). If they leave and then can't get another job they may file for unemployment and if you have not paid unemployment tax as an employer out of their paychecks, you may be responsible to do so, even 5 years down the road. You may also be held liable for backlogged state and federal taxes. My suggestion is to set up a payroll with your bank that will cover all of this. It will be a bit more expensive than paying out of your pocket privately but it will give you piece of mind. Do not pay under the table no matter what – you will get burned.

How do you pay an employee?

You must pay at least the federal minimum wage; currently in MA is $7.25 per hour. If your employee is not an independent contractor and/or lives out of the home, overtime for any hours over 40 must be paid. Overtime is time and a half. If your employee is in a salary position, and that position is agreed upon over 40 hours in a week, it must be very clearly stated the hours expected for the salary position and what rate overtime will be paid and when (the hourly rate must still be at least $7.25 for a salary employee). You should look at the Fair Labor Standards Act to check your states minimum wage. You should also check the Companionship Services act in the FLSA for a salary employee especially if you have them working unto or over 60 hours a week. You should set up a payment plan with your bank so that all taxes are taken out and you are not stuck paying after the fact. You must pay your FICA taxes. Typically, each party (employer/employee) contributes 7.65%; however, if the family fails to collect this tax via payroll deductions from the employee, the family will be liable for both the employer and employee portion of the tax. Simply put, if your aide takes off and then you are paying your taxes she/he's not responsible for their part – you double up on the payment. You must pay workman's comp in the state of MA (check your state to see if you do also).

Forms: you keep the original and give an executed copy to your aide. Please, please protect yourself! All of these forms can be easily downloaded from online free legal sites. You can also just make up your own (check examples on the web). They don't need to be fancy but they do need to be signed and dated by both parties (whoever is employing the aide and the aide).

Employee time sheet:
Of course you will be able to tell who was where and when via the journal that they are keeping but it will be a pain to put it all together, just keep a clip board with photo copied time sheets and have each aide fill them out at the beginning and end of each shift. Only allow 15-minute increments to save your sanity to avoid adding everything up. Designate a day and place in the home for the timesheets to be left. Specify that there should be no overlap in time. For example: *aide comes in for a shift at 8 p.m. to relieve the day aide, but the day aide puts down that she stayed until 8:15 p.m.; there is a 15-minute time overlap. This should never be the case. Assuming everyone is on time the shift should end/start on schedule, if an aide stays to chat on her own time that is her own time. This should be made clear. It may seem like a little thing but the cost will add up over time and if allowed (or ignored) it might be taken advantage of.
Name | Date | Time in | Time out| Total time
Liability release form:
Is your aide going to drive your cared for (if so, make sure to put them on YOUR insurance). Are they going to run errands for them on their own time? Really brainstorm this one, everything and anything should go on here. Do you have a dog that is a bit snappy, a pool that someone could slip by? Driving is a BIG one. Unless there is a lot of driving daily my suggestion is to take a taxi service. If you must have the aide drive, make sure that you are paying the additional coverage on her/your insurance to cover your cared one. In addition, have them sign a release of liability should there be an accident.

Employee Warning letter:
You need to give one verbal and two written warnings before you can fire someone and be pretty sure they will not come back and sue you. MA will state which technically means that anyone can be let go or leave at any point for any reason. However, if you want to fight unemployment you will need to have a track record of non-compliance in addition to a signed agreement listing the rules to show that a) they were provided the rules and b) signed off on them c) the rules were broken resulting in termination as was previously stated would happen.

Employment agreement:
This is probably the most important. The employee agreement can be as simple or as complicated as you want to make it, but it is the document that will bind your agreement. Make sure to have a detailed job description attached to this, and ensure that it is signed and dated. Make sure to note the hours, rate/salary agreed upon, W9 etc. In addition, at the end of this workbook is a sample handbook. You should read through and alter where you need to, but this is something to attach to the employee agreement that should cover a lot of the bases.

Notes:

Independent Contractor form (instead or in addition to the job application). Make sure you are actually hiring an independent contractor (20 questions listed below). Have the prospective employer provide you with evidence of business credentials and insurance, such as articles of incorporation and insurance policies.

20 questions Independent Contractors should answer yes to:

1. Are you required to comply with instructions about when, where, and how the work is to be done? (No.)
2. Does your client provide you with training to enable you to perform a job in a particular method or manner? (No.)
3. Are the services you provide integrated into your client's business operation? (No.)
4. Must the services be rendered by you personally? (No.)
5. Do you have the capability to hire, supervise, or pay assistants to help you in performing the services under contract? (Yes.)
6. Is the relationship between you and the person or company you perform services for a continuing relationship? (No.)
7. Who sets the hours of work? (You do.)
8. Are you required to devote your full time to the person or company you perform services for? (No.)
9. Is the work performed at the place of business of the potential employer? (No.)
10. Who directs the order or sequence in which the work must be done? (You do.)
11. Are you required to provide regular written or oral reports to your client? (No.)
12. What is the method of payment — hourly, commission or by the job? (Contingency or project milestone-based payments are ideal.)
13. Are your business and/or traveling expenses reimbursed? (No.)
14. Who furnishes tools and materials used in providing services? (You do.)
15. Do you have a significant investment in facilities used to perform services? (Yes. The more substantial your investment, the better.)
16. Can you realize both a profit and a loss? (Yes.)
17. Can you work for a number of firms at the same time? (Yes.)
18. Do you make your services available to the general public? (Yes. It's a good idea to have a business listing in the phone book, for example.)
19. Are you subject to dismissal for reasons other than nonperformance of contract Specifications? (No. In addition, your client should provide at least a week's notice. Termination at
    will makes you look like an employee.)
20. Can you terminate your relationship without incurring a liability for failure to complete a job? (Yes, assuming you're working on a time-and-materials basis. If you're working on a project, or milestone, basis, you are obligated to deliver on your commitments if you wish to be paid for your efforts.)

Notes:

Employment Application: all the information you legally can require including references etc.

Authority to release employment information:
Should someone call you with a reference check etc. you want authority to release this information or you're breaking the law.

Verification of education form: *you may want to ask for a copy of the graduate degree from their schools but it's a personal choice. Verification of Licensure form: copy front and back the HHA/CNA license and make note of expiration date and note they will be responsible for renewing their license).

Employment eligibility verification form:
If you have someone out of the country you need a license, passport with a work permit (in date – keep track of when it expires) or SS #.

Work Injury report:
This will be provided by your insurance company: multiple copies of the workman's work injury reports should be kept in the house in a designated spot. The aide should be instructed in writing at any point if she/he incurs an injury while working. They must immediately fill out a report and call the point person. The point person will then call your insurance agency (within 24hrs or time allotted by insurance policy) and report the injury. This is very important so the story doesn't change after the fact.

A few side notes I just think are helpful…

Personal Safety: There are all sorts of safety devices out there. From first alert 'I've fallen and I can't get up', to floor mats that alarm should someone get out of bed in the middle of the night, rails by the toilet / bathtub for stability, urinals / commodes for easy transfers during the evening…it's worth a look. If you have a 'sleeping aide' which you pay her/him for sleeping but being on alert you will want to have a foot mat so that it alarms when the cared for gets out of bed, people will forget to ring the bells and then there's risk of a fall.

Personal Hygiene:
Gloves, sanitizer, pull-ups for inconstancies, bed mats for incontinent persons, a seasoned aide will tell you exactly what is needed. Alternatively, ask a training center for advice or an evaluation.
Connect to websites who will send you monthly newsletters that, for example, will focus on things to watch out for in the wintertime, what are the new elderly fraud (usually door-to-door sales or flyers etc.)…as I said, once this is set up you have to maintain it

Veteran's assistance: The United States Congress passed a special pension for veterans in 1951. This allows seniors tax-free money to pay their expenses, protect assets/income and could offset costs of LTC. The benefit is great. A veteran with a dependent may receive up to $1,949.00 per month. A veteran alone may receive up to $1,644.00 per month or a surviving spouse may receive up to $1,056.00 per month. The benefits are tax-free and are deposited EFT just like Social Security. If you call Veterans Angels, Inc. (it's all free) they will help you with the application. 888-319-1117.

If you have a **Long Term Health (LTC)** plan you will have to prove the payments that have been made in order to be reimbursed. As long as we're talking about LTC, what they usually ask for reimbursement is a copy of the work log (notebook kept by aides) and a copy of the payment receipts or invoices (if you had the aide invoice you – but this is usually a time sheet). All LTC programs are different; make sure you find out exactly what they need and when they need it, so you can be reimbursed, in writing. In my experience they are notorious for saying your check will go out on such a date and then it is three months later.

The following duties are typically not approved for aides. If you need/want these activities you should specify them in your work agreement/handbook and a release of liability so that the aide cannot sue you:

> May not change a dressing nor apply solutions or ointment to a wound dressing.
>
> May not assist with tube feeding.
>
> May not irrigate a foley catheter.
>
> May not irrigate a colostomy through a stoma.
>
> May not give any kind of enema.
>
> May not dis-impact a rectum.
>
> May not give medications, including pills, eye drops, liquid medications, rectal suppositories;   may only offer medication.
>
> May not perform chest physical therapy or postural drainage.
>
> May not change IV bags or touch the dials of any IV machine.
>
> May not cut toenails at any time.
>
> May not carry an adult person or large child at any time.
>
> May not do heavy housework like washing windows, floors etc.
>
> May not drive a in his/her own car, the car or any other car.
>
> May not cash a checks or lottery tickets or use the _____ ATM or credit cards.
>
> May not smoke in the home.

Checklist: Communication – documentation –execution
- ✓ Family meeting
- ✓ Build your family responsibility schedule and have key dates to check in with each other
- ✓ Start to build your model – what is the daily/weekly routine, behaviors, likes, dislikes, favorite foods, time up and to bed, time of medication, how many times does the care for get up during the night, are they stable, what could you do to make things easier etc.
- ✓ Start to build your work agreement based upon the above

- ✓ Start to build the daily/weekly/monthly schedule (always keep a calendar in the home for appointments etc.)
- ✓ Build your schedule: mornings, afternoons, and evenings…overnight, daytime?
- ✓ Look for aides – start to interview etc.
- ✓ Hire and keep a close eye, make changes as needed immediately
- ✓ Keep a copy of the handbook in the home
- ✓ Start a notebook for all aides to complete during their shifts in an on-time manner
- ✓ You could also hire on a temp to hire bases, so that there is a trial period before immediate hire…
- ✓ Maintain, maintain, maintain

If you have read this and you are still at a loss, here's a tip far too often overlooked: you can hire geriatric care managers (GCM), whom are often medical professionals and/or counselors who have taken an alternative route as a consultant. A GCM will come in to your home and do a complete evaluation and help you step by step. You will pay for this service but they will save you time and set you up and then you will be in charge of running it. If you're dealing with setting up nutritionists, physical therapists or extreme obstacles to safe living etc. it's not a bad idea to at least have a meeting with a GCM in your area so that you have a contact to connect with when you have a question that you don't have an answer to or if you need recommendations.

Good luck!

If you would like to contact me directly to discuss personal consulting please email me mappingprivatecare@gmail.com

Notes:

Example Handbook outline:

Introduction:

This handbook is intended to serve as a practical guide to _____ personal policies and practices and is relevant to all of _____ employees. However, since it is only a summary compiled for your convenience, it is not intended to cover all topics or circumstances and reserves the right to respond to specific situations as necessary. _____ reserves the right to revise, amend, add, and/or delete policies and procedures. As new policies are developed, and outdated policies are modified or deleted to deal with new situations, conditions, or laws, we _____ will attempt to inform employees of changes in policies. The policies in this handbook, however, may change without notice.

<u>Guidelines and employee responsibilities:</u>

Please remember that it is the right of _____ to have all information both medical and personal kept confidential. A breach of this rule will lead to immediate dismissal.

_____ is your number one priority

There is no sleeping on any shifts unless otherwise specified in your shift agreement.

_____ is to be bathed daily or according to care plan.

_____ that are incontinent should be checked at the beginning of each shift and regularly throughout, minimally every 2 hours; do not leave it for somebody else to do. Each time a diaper is changed, you are required to wash _____ thoroughly to prevent rashes and bedsores.

_____ is to be repositioned hourly unless otherwise instructed.

Protective gloves must be worn when in contact with or handling body secretions or drainage. They must always be changed after handling body secretions or drainage and hands washed. New gloves should then be reapplied the next time you engage in an activity requiring the contact with body secretions or drainage. Do not wear gloves outside the areas of direct use (i.e. the bathroom).

Notebooks must be kept during and completed at the end of each shift and must accurately reflect the work completed on an hourly basis.

If _____ does not respond when you arrive at their home and you are unable to gain admittance you must call _____ immediately. Carry the _____ and office telephone numbers at all times in case of an emergency.

Call _____ the aide on duty if you are going to be late. Make sure to reflect this in your timesheet. If the aide cannot stay on to wait for you or there is no aide there, call
.

Time sheets are due every _____ (day) _____ by _____ (time) _____. Please complete your time sheet and leave it in the designated spot on the last day of the week you are working.

Schedule and Attendance

- If you want to change your shift or schedule temporarily or permanently you must notify_____of the request to change as soon as possible, even if it is a fair shift exchange with another aide.

If you want to request time off you must do so at least 2 weeks in advance to allow proper coverage to be arranged.

Employee Responsibilities:

Inform your family and friends that you may not receive personal phone calls at work except in the event of an emergency.

Take personal pride in your appearance.

Assist new employees by making them feel welcome and be helpful with their questions/training.

Report any violation of policy or other problems to _____.

Supply your own meals while on shift. Groceries at _____ home are for - _____and bought on _____ budget.

Professional Conduct and Personal Appearance:

The appearance and conduct of staff members reflects upon you directly. All employees are expected to maintain excellent hygiene, report to work in approved upon attire that allows range and motion for duties, and to conduct themselves in a professional manner, which respects the privacy, reputation and wellbeing of _____.

Aide activities:

Bathing: bed, tub, shower or sponge

Care of hair: combing, brushing and shampoo

Care of skin: fingernails and shaving

Care of mouth: teeth and dentures

Toileting and use of bedpans and urinals

Transferring in and out of bed into a chair, toilet or commode

Assist with use of Hoyer lift and other transfer equipment

Assist ambulation with cane, crutches and walker

Dressing and undressing

Feeding

Positioning in bed or chair for comfortable body posture

Range of motion exercises and assisting with rehabilitation activities

Taking and recording temperature, pulse and respiration

Measuring and recording intake and output

Applying non-prescription cream or solution to an unopened area

Perform Household services:

Light housekeeping, specifically:

Laundry for the_____.

Meal preparation (including special diets).

Clean up after meals, washing dishes for/by the_____.

Making and changing the occupied/unoccupied bed.

Remind _____to take medicine.

Assist the _____with divisional activities (i.e. playing cards, board games etc.).

Weigh _____ in the AM/PM and record the weight in the notebook.

If physical, mental and behavioral changes in the client should be noted immediately and then documented in the notebook.

<u>The following is cause for immediate dismissal/ Prohibited administrative conduct:</u>

1. Claims for payment or reimbursement of any kind that are false, fraudulent, inaccurate or fictitious

2. Falsified medical records, time cards or any other record used as the basis for submitting claims

3. Using the clients phone for personal calls

4. Excessive absences and /or tardiness in reporting to work

5. Behavior not deemed appropriate for the workplace

6. Failing to carry out assigned responsibilities

7. Leaving the assigned without permission

8. Failing to promptly report a job related incident such as an injury or unusual occurrence

9. Soliciting or accepting gifts

10. Conducting personal business or enterprise in the home

11. Stealing property and/or unauthorized personal use of possession of property

12. Deliberately mistreating or displaying negligence with may result in injury

13. Sleeping during work hours

14. Coming to work under the influence of alcohol or illegal drugs. Refusing to be tested for alcohol or drug use if there is reasonable cause to suspect such influence

15. Insubordination, including, but not limited to open defiance of instruction from _____ or _____, and/or neglect of care plan duties

16. Forging, altering, or deliberately falsifying any document, authorization, record, employment application or time card. Making fraudulent or misleading statements of any kind

17. Engaging in unlawful, indecent, or immoral conduct on property during or outside work hours. Conviction of a felony or other criminal charges. Failure to report any suspicious, unethical or illegal conduct by fellow employees, residents or vendors

18. Job Abandonment: an employee who fails to report to work without notifying _____ (no call/no show) or an employee who fails to return from an approved Leave of Absence at the approved return date will be deemed to have abandoned and terminated his or her job

19. Loud, angry or disruptive behavior that is not part of the typical work environment

20. Commission of a felony or misdemeanor on property

21. Any other conduct that a reasonable person would perceive as constituting a threat of violence

22. Discussion of personal financial issues

23. Acceptance of money or gifts from _____

24. Discussion of confidential matters pertaining to _____ family, legal, financial privacy

25. Smoking on property

Termination of Employment:

Voluntary Resignation: initiated in writing by the employee to_____ with a requested minimum of two weeks working notice. Failure to give and work adequate notice without extenuating circumstances may result in disqualification for rehire.

Termination: when an employee is discharged for violation of work agreement, policies and procedures.

Discipline:

_____requires compliance with basic policies and rules to insure the safety and well-being of_____. Actions by employees that are not in the best interest of the welfare of_____may result in appropriate disciplinary actions, including termination of employment. At its sole discretion,   may use the following disciplinary procedure or any part of the following procedure for disciplinary actions: verbal warning, written warning and termination.

Verbal warnings are designed to encourage correction of the undesirable behavior or unsatisfactory performance. A verbal warning does not need to be signed; however, a documentation of this warning will be kept in the employee personal file

Written warnings must be signed by both parties and will be kept in the file

Termination will be executed if the offense is serious enough to excuse the employee immediately due to liability of character and/or job performance. In very serious cases no written or verbal warning has to be given